Bedtime Procrastination Cure

Beat Social Jetlag, become an early riser, conquer insomnia, sleep well & live an energetic life

Dylan Johnson

Table of Contents

Introduction

Modern living has granted us many luxuries. We control our indoor climates; have information available 24/7 by touching glowing rectangles to consume infinite volumes of entertainment. The flipside is that nobody put in an 'off' switch in our heads to let us stop consumption at any time. Work and play just stream to the average person in one giant, amorphous torrent via smart phones, social networks and screens of different sizes. The currency we use to pay for this high availability of technology is usually in "hours of sleep". We intuitively know about the importance of sleep but never seem to be able to prioritize it high enough to take action and correct an errant bedtime schedule. There is this terrible domino effect of problems that accumulate over a long period of poor sleep habits. Are you one of those people who consider themselves a night owl? Do you envy people who seem to wake up early every morning and look well put together? Do you constantly live with regret or guilt the next day after sleeping too late and having to get up earlier and groggier for work or school? This book is written for you.

Bedtime procrastination is one of those problems that would not have existed prior to the invention of television. Netflix, Snapchat and email have only made things worse. There are very few explicit options for a person crippled by bedtime procrastination or social jetlag. The behaviors are automatic and even medical professionals tend to commonly dismiss symptoms as generally insomnia related. In fact the broad causes of bedtime procrastination are largely a combination bad habits, psychological issues and impulse control. Every person seems to have a different array of factors contributing to the problem making it very difficult for sleep experts to come up with a formula to address it. In this book, you will gain concrete insights into what causes your automatic behaviors and thought processes leading to poor sleep schedules. Some of them will be obvious and some will be more obscure. Awareness is the key to beating poor sleep related behavior. We will also be going through some very specific things you can do to improve the odds of you sleeping on time and with a regular pattern. Follow through with the advice and you will see your sleep patterns normalize. Like any persistent negative behavior, it will take commitment and work. Power through with the techniques and you will see many areas of your life streamline itself. The benefits are absolutely worth it. Your health, relationships and mental health will improve if your sleep is sound, regular, predictable and restful.

The insights in this book have been collected through experience from working with clients who have complained of out of the ordinary sleep timing issues. I have a unique insight into what are practical approaches to fixing a sleep pattern. Many of my clients have either completely reset their sleep cycles or significantly improved the timing and quality of their sleep. My techniques are unorthodox and have not been discussed in mainstream literature on the subject but give them a go and you are sure to see results. Consider this an intervention – you need to sleep on time and wake up early to be successful in life. Congratulations on taking your first step towards a lifestyle where well timed bedtime patterns are an automatic part of your life. Soon you will feel rested, energized and ready to conquer life. In my experience, this could be the one factor holding you back from achieving your dreams.

Hello Night Owl

If you are a night owl, the good news is that you don't have to feel bad about sleeping late. A 1998 sleep habit study done at the University of England concluded that there was no evidence about going to bed and waking up early having any associated benefit on health, socioeconomic or cognitive function. On the contrary, the night owls showed a noticeable wealth and intelligence advantage over the early risers in the study group. Does this mean you should close this book and go back to your late night sleep habits? You shouldn't because the reason you picked up this book is most likely due to the fact that the world and society functions in a way that benefits early risers. Work schedules start early in the morning, school tends to begin early in the day, McDonalds has that wonderful breakfast menu only till 10 AM. This makes early birds happier in general when compared to night owls. It is possible to use the techniques in this book and remain consistent enough to retain the intelligence advantages you most likely have from being a night owl while still being respected by society as an early bird who gets the worm. On the flip side, night owls also tend to be partial to bad habits like smoking and drinking. Becoming an early riser would likely result in an improvement in healthier habits like exercise while also decreasing activity from negative areas because night life tends to be more conducive to drinking and smoking. You most likely harbor beliefs related to delayed sleep times that prevent you from altering your sleep schedule e.g. late sleepers are creative people. The goal is not to make you a boring person but to achieve balance in your life. The amazing things that happen once you reverse a poor sleep trend are nothing short of incredible. No amount of self-help seminars or psychedelic drugs can have that dramatic an impact on your life. I've seen night owl executives who had conquered the corporate ladder's major challenges but feared an early morning meeting. Don't sleepwalk through your life. Take action and ensure that you get enough sleep from a regular sleep cycle. You are a binary being who has two states – sleep and wakefulness. These two phases need to be in balance for you to function optimally. Procrastination of your bedtime will never allow the necessary balance to be achieved.

Procrastination

There are 3 key reasons why you procrastinate in general:

1. Feeling forced to do the activity (feeling compelled, not feeling you have control)

2. Not having enough faith in your ability to do the activity (fearing failure)

3. Not having enough reason to do the activity (a lack of purpose)

The first thing to do would be to reflect upon which of the above reasons apply to your sleep patterns. Ask yourself questions. Write down your thoughts on the topic. Later on in this book, I will be introducing the concept of a sleep journal. For now, the best thing to do would be to maintain an exclusive journal to jot down thoughts related to resistance to sleep. Chronic bedtime procrastinators usually face some combination of the 3 reasons. Flesh them out in your journal and ponder the points you come up with. This activity alone will set the stage for you to conquer sleep issues.

Follow these guidelines to beat your tendency to procrastinate sleep:

Plan: plan your sleep goals out. Now that you have a high level understanding of what might be driving your poor sleep habits, it's time to start some high level planning. An amorphous goal is not going to help so you need to write down some reasonable goals including timelines and approaches to reach this goal. As you progress you can refine these goals but the act of planning in itself would involve chunking this broad sleep goal into smaller, more manageable activities. Determine your optimal bed time. Define a rational sleep window. Be as realistic as possible and write down a plan on how you might gradually improve your bedtime by just 15 minutes a week for 4 weeks that would lead to your perfect sleep cycle. Remember that if you slept 15 minutes earlier you have to also wake up a corresponding 15 minutes earlier. Also try to pencil in corresponding time shifts in correlated activities like taking a shower or brushing your teeth. In your initial goal setting, don't worry too much about whether you completely achieve them or not but do your best to stay consistent with your new habit modifications. Living life according to a strict schedule is boring and impractical. This is just a start and you will not need to follow a schedule after your initial planning month. Real progress will be made if you chip away at the problem so it's important to temper expectations so that you don't expect too much at the beginning of your journey.

Just do it: When your set bedtime hits, you need to take action and just stop what you are doing and go to bed. Sure it's easier said than done but if you can somehow just stop what you are doing (like binge watching a show on Netflix) and get ready for bed, you will in time be able to build momentum and thought control to the point where it becomes easier and easier to just get up and go back to bed. Enough wins in this area will really improve your self esteem and encourage you to do the right thing when the time gets close to your optimal bedtime.

Create an impetus: write down (in your sleep journal) how your life would be if you had this sleep issue for the next 5 years without improvement. Reflect on what issues you might face. Do the same thing by projecting how having poor sleep habits will affect your ten years from now with zero improvement. This part of the activity is not pleasant but once you are done projecting 10 years into the future, close your eyes and visualize how you would feel 1 year from now if you had solved this sleep pattern. What are the goals you might achieve? Would you feel healthier? Would you feel less guilt? Would there be less fear in your life? Write these thoughts down after you swim in the bliss of how good things would be if you didn't have these issues. Do the same thing by projecting 5 years and 10 years into the future where sleep patterns are no longer an issue for you. The goal is to create contrast and eliminate procrastination reason number 3 i.e. not having enough reason to correct your sleep patterns.

We are going to get into more specific techniques and insights to address your social jetlag and bedtime procrastination but remember to finish the above exercise to get some momentum going before we get into the next section.

Bedtime Procrastination & Social Jetlag

When it comes to bedtime procrastination, there may be more at work than just general procrastination mechanisms. This peculiar behavior is very common and damaging obviously because sufferers put off bedtime even if they are very tired. The long term implications of poor sleep on both physical and mental health are enormous. You are gaining weight, feeling more anxious and losing attention span because of poor sleep patterns. Fixing this behavior is going to help you turn your life around. If you are a bedtime procrastinator you will find yourself going to bed later than you wanted at least a few times a week. That is a unique aspect of bedtime procrastinators. They tend to have a mental deadline for what time they would like to sleep but never seem to achieve that time.

Social Jetlag is a related condition where the sleep issue is related to different sleep patterns on weekends versus the rest of the work week. Social Jetlag is a disorder related to modern living. It's very common for people to sleep in on weekends after going to bed late. Weekend nights also usually involve going out, socializing, increased social media usage and partying. Binge watching or video games tend to also feature prominently on weekend schedules. Monday morning however requires a return to the original sleep pattern with an early start. Your body is simply not designed to constantly shift sleep patterns so rapidly and hence an effect similar to jet lag is experienced. There is a strong causal link between obesity and social jetlag. Social jetlag is related to bedtime procrastination in that people who follow a pattern leading to social jetlag would have a strong tendency to postpone sleep during weekdays thereby leading to extremely short sleep durations during the work or study week. The associated grogginess from this lifestyle disease has a tremendous impact on work productivity. If you feel depressed at work, try fixing your sleep patterns first before exploring options like switching careers. Relationships also tend to suffer from chronic sleep patterns like social jetlag because couples tend to influence each other's sleep habits. A couple who suffers from social jetlag together could develop relationship issues related to the poor judgment associated with mental exhaustion. The point is that this is not some minor issue related to modern living in the first world. It's a ticking time bomb that is sapping everybody of health and productivity. Unfortunately, it is common for even some medical professionals to dismiss the severity of bedtime procrastination and social jetlag or to address these issues the same way you would address conventional insomnia. Companies, colleges and schools also have not caught up to the latest in sleep science to bake in flexibility and mechanisms to address these issues. There is this terrible message conveyed in many tv shows and movies related to company, corporate or college culture; that a dedicated worker or student is one who doesn't get much sleep. That popular cop drama usually shows the detective drinking coffee in every scene and making a point about how little they slept the previous night; the lawyer in the latest legal drama will talk about how they stayed up 'all night' with the case files. This is not a badge of honor. Every time you see a message like that being conveyed in the media that you consume, you should view those characters as flawed and unwise. The lawyer would probably be more productive on the case if they managed to pace themselves working through the case files and still getting a decent amount of sleep. Science shows the exact opposite as being more effective.

Nudging versus nagging

A common tendency for people addressing a bad habit is to attempt to power through with raw will power and try and hammer the unwanted behavior into submission. This inevitably sets one up for failure as it is perceived by the mind as a 'nag' and mental processes to resist this nag will kick in. Think about when you were a child or a teenager and were grounded. Sending you to your room was something you did not want to do but had to. Martial artists understand at a physical level, that one should not try to resist incoming force from their opponent but instead use the opponent's force against them. Similarly, you must ease yourself into a better sleep routine rather than attempt to brute force your way into the right rhythm. The preferred mindset you must have is a 'nudging' mindset to allow easing into better sleep hygiene. You can nudge your sleep patterns back to normal by improving your sleep time by 15 minutes every 2 days for instance. Make a list of activities performed on an average day before going to bed. Then start working on nudging each sleep precursor activity's time earlier by 15 minutes. By brushing your teeth 15 minutes sooner for instance, you will free up enough bandwidth to sleep earlier.

While it may seem obvious, many bedtime procrastinators mismanage their time in activities prior to sleep either unknowingly or with intent to push their bedtime further away because they might not look forward to the following day's activities as contrasted against their current 'fun' time. Let's get into some specific techniques around how you can regularize your sleep patterns and pay off that sleep debt.

Technique 1: Optimize weekend sleep patterns

If your problem is social jetlag, then the first line of defense would be to work on normalizing your weekend sleep patterns. Your weekends should not be that different from your weekdays from a bedtime and wake up time perspective. Easier said than done because most of us use the weekend to unwind. Social jetlag is the equivalent of what a globetrotting executive feels when they constantly wake up in a different global time zone. As you might expect, many individuals who travel that regularly face enormous health and mental challenges in the long term. Rockstars and global DJs on tour tend to cope with their professionally induced social jetlag usually with substance abuse or alcohol. As we have seen, the tendency to sleep later has a correlation with substance abuse habits.

Sleep logic: If you can mentally shift your view of the weekend from being this once in a lifetime type occurrence and be pragmatic about sleep patterns, the social jetlag will not affect you as much. The most common mistake people make on the weekend is not setting an alarm to wake up on a weekend morning. Sleeping in on the weekend is a very bad habit that will negatively impact the time you go to bed at later on. Napping during the day on the weekend is another big mistake. Yes, power naps have been shown in many studies to improve performance and genuinely improve energy levels but for a chronic bedtime procrastinator or someone suffering from social jetlag, naps will only make the problem worse. If you absolutely must nap, keep it under ten minutes but my recommendation is to stay away from napping completely.

I'm definitely not recommending you give up your social life completely but becoming aware of the implications of a completely boundary less weekend existence is what is going to improve the quality of your life and reduce the impact of social jetlag. Planning out your sleep patterns in advance so that you are able to drift back to a bedtime closer to what you would require on Sunday night to be fresh on Monday morning is going to go a long way in reducing the impact of a late night out on Friday or Saturday night.

Technique 2: Smart Alarm Systems

Everyone is familiar with setting an alarm clock or setting an alarm on their phone to wake up but what should be done in order to promote better sleep habits is an alarm to remind you to go to bed. Changing the way you use alarms in your life is going to change your perception of alarms as this dreadful mechanism that jolts you out of sleep to something more meaningful as a nudge. Once you have identified and noted down sleep precursor activities, set an alarm on your phone long enough in advance to allow you to stop whatever activity you were doing and prepare to go to bed. You have to stay diligent with this alarm system and really take the deadline seriously. This means that if the sleep alarm goes off when you're in the middle of a gripping episode of your Netflix TV show, you will have to be disciplined enough to hit the off switch. The initial week would be the hardest but sticking with the program particularly in cases like a TV show binge watching bender or an unstoppable 'Call of duty' session. Try to rationalize how the video game that you are playing or the TV show that you are watching will remain the next day and afterwards as well. Ideally your sleep alarm should go off at a time optimal to allow getting some closure on whatever entertainment you might be consuming that evening. If the primary activity you pursue every evening relates to work, then try and set an email deadline time linked to your alarm after which you will not check or reply to emails.

When waking up every morning, I highly recommend you switch alarm clock technologies to newer options that allow waking you up in a gentler manner. Apps like 'Sleep Cycle' allow installing smart alarm clocks on your phone that can be placed on your nightstand which then wakes you up in your lightest sleep phase. This simple shift in the way you wake up will have a dramatic effect on your sleep and the sensations you have upon first waking up every mroning. Device companies like Withings also make smart alarms clocks and sleep sensors that can improve your sleep. If you want to wake up in a gentler fashion and don't want to use sound or don't want to wake up your partner, a fitness band with sleep tracking ability should work well for you. Smart fitness trackers from Fitbit and Jawbone have gentle vibrating alarms that will quietly wake you up. Later on in this book, I will also show you how to use light based alarm clocks to wake up totally refreshed and energized. Your key take away from this section should be about using technology to positively enhance your sleep and wake up patterns. Stop using a noisy alarm to jar you out of deep REM sleep leading to a terrible day.

Technique 3: Entertainment Replacement

I've seen a number of people fall into the trap of consuming on demand cable or Netflix type services all day long but if you have a desire to really excel at life and achieve your goals, you might want to combine your sleep optimization efforts with daily rituals and activities that enrich you and take you closer to a powerful lifestyle. For my clients who feel a desire to really take their general performance to the next level, I always recommend replacing an amount of television show consumption with reading. I can't stress enough how powerful reading can be as a means to really transform yourself. There's something about the consumption of information in that format that beats Youtube videos, Twitter and Netflix any day of the week. Millennials are particularly at risk of losing that long term reading habit. Choose books that you find interesting and try to read regularly every day. Kindles have made this activity easy and enjoyable. Making reading a daily activity will also have a tremendous effect on your sleep routine. Reading every day, even on a Kindle will reduce your exposure to **blue light**. Modern LED type displays emit high amounts of blue light. Smartphones, laptops and tablets are all negatively impacting your sleep due to the amount of blue light emitted by them straight into the sensitive receptors in your eyes. Darkness or the absence of blue light is a natural cue to your system that it's time to sleep. As cave people, humans used to sleep based on the time that the sun rose and set. Nowadays, to our internal clocks there is no distinct difference between day and night. Switching to a physical book at night or reading off a Kindle can help you rediscover natural sleepiness at night time. Reading will also make you a better, more knowledgeable and articulate person. If you are not a natural reader, the best way to create a reading habit would be to gradually ease yourself into it by reading a little bit every day. Treat a few pages the way you would treat a Tumblr post. Like a good cardio program, you will notice your capacity to read increase as you become more consistent with the practice. Choosing to read fiction just before sleeping is a great option because reading fiction can help switch off the critical, judgmental portion of your mind allowing you to sleep and dream deeper. Obviously reading intense fiction novels could have the equivalent mental effect of watching a

Michael Bay movie so choose the fiction books you read with care. Fiction is also a great way to keep reading as a fun activity. A heavy, non-fiction book is more likely to discourage you from reading in general or remind you of boring times at school before a midterm.

Technique 4: Digital Detox

If you have the willpower to improve your sleep patterns, that's great. All you have to do is follow through with the positive nudging steps I've outlined above to improve your life. The issue that many people face in modern times is the constant availability of distractions. Your smart phone is always available at a moment's notice to engulf you in a stream of constant distractions and dopamine rushes. I recommend that people with self-regulation issues related to tablet or iPhone use browse the app store for apps that enable automated preset locking of devices to limit their use and prevent you from getting distracted from more productive activities like going to sleep. Search the app store for keywords like procrastination, phone lock, etc. to find apps that address this issue. Flipd and Cold turkey are two apps that serve this purpose quite well. First identify the specific digital distraction and then research the technique that can be used to restrict usage in the evening or at bedtime. Windows laptops for instance come with a built in task scheduling option that allows you to define a shutdown time every day. Talk to a computer repair expert if you think this mechanism could benefit you. If you have a roommate, spouse or friend who can intervene at a specified time to make you switch off your PS4 or whatever device keeps you up at night, which will be far easier than a technology led intervention.

I had a client with a bad habit of listening to pounding electronic music every evening after coming home from work. I noticed that he had a strong passion for this type of music (I'm more of a Rolling Stones fan) but I saw the value he received from relaxing after work by playing his favorite music really loud. The problem was that he wouldn't let the music die down and would only stop playing the music when it was absolutely time to go to bed. The result was that his mind was way too wired and alert to fall asleep after getting such a loud dose of pulsating music. I had him resolve this by simply switching his time for music enjoyment to the morning when he would work out. Sometimes the simplest of solutions can have the greatest impact. Analyze your digital usage and then institute measures to control their use. I'm not a big fan of outright denial. Denial breeds resistance in the long run and besides isn't the point of modern living to utilize technology effectively to improve our lives?

In addition to using apps that prevent phone usage, it would also be worthwhile in using apps to cut out blue light emanating from phone, laptop and tablet screens. Search the app store for 'blue light' and you will find many apps that filter out the blue light from your device. F.lux is a free application for laptops that allow blue light to be filtered out depending on the time of the day. Certain televisions and devices like the Saffron Drift come with a feature for blue light filtering. If you use these technologies in addition to your daily viewing habits, you can rebalance your response to light. The easiest hack to filter out blue light would be to buy blue blocking glasses. Many options exist for amber colored lenses that filter out blue light. Optometrists are familiar with this requirement and speaking to them to get a pair will be worth it in the long run because there is simply no way we can eliminate digital devices from our lives completely. I've reviewed some specific apps and technologies to address bedtime procrastination on my blog at sleepquation.com

Technique 5: Sleep Environment Preparation

If your bedroom is not conducive to sleep, then you will inevitably develop poor sleep habits and patterns. Sleep, like all other activities needs to be compelling enough for you to respect the cycle. Some of the more obvious measures that need to be taken involve keeping your bed only for sleep and sex. This advice is old but solid. Some of the worst habits related to sleep involve watching TV in bed or using your smart phone lying down. You want to create a strong association between your bed and sleep. Ensure that your bed is cool and comfortable enough. Sometimes, even expensive sheets can make a bed retain too much heat, making it uncomfortable for deep sleep. Choosing sheets that have a cool touch to them will help you sleep better.

Improving air: Temperature is not the only factor in sleeping well. If you snore or suffer from sleep apnea, a simple hack to improve the quality of your sleep would be to use a humidifier or vaporizer. Depending on where you live, humidity levels could be low and dry air is much more difficult to breathe in through your nostrils when you sleep. Moisturizing the air in such a situation using a humidifier could have a dramatic impact on the quality of your sleep. You should ideally pick up a humidity monitor and use it to determine if you require a humidifier or a dehumidifier (if your room features too much moisture). Living in a city would also mean poor indoor air quality. Investing in a quality air purifier would enhance your bedroom's air quality thereby making you wake up feeling rested further encouraging your efforts to improve sleep patterns.

Controlling light: Our bodies are designed to react to light. It goes without saying that our eyes and even the cells we are made up of have specialized receptors to react to light. You should ideally be sleeping in a very dark environment; pitch black if possible so that your nervous system understands the difference between day and night further improving your sleep pattern. If you don't already have blackout curtains, investing in them would be the first thing you should do. Using black tape to mask bright electronic indicator lights on devices also works great. My own cell phone has a notification light that was really messing with my sleep. I found a setting to disable the annoying little light but placing your phone in a desk drawer would also work. Fluorescent & LED lighting really wreck your natural circadian rhythms. In order to offset the bad effects of modern lighting systems, I highly recommend you use **red spectrum light**. Certain spectrums of red light have positive effects on collagen production, meaning your skin would look better in the long run and there is some evidence of certain red spectrum lights improving beneficial hormone levels. You do not need an expensive light machine to achieve this. You can get regular red LED strip lighting used for Christmas on Amazon. Having a few strips of that in your bedroom or in a room where you have fluorescent lighting or a television and other sources of blue light will offset the negative effects of the blue spectrum light. Aside from regular strip lighting, you can also invest in smart bulbs or smart home devices like the Philips hue lighting system. Smart bulbs sometimes come with configurable color settings that can sometimes be controlled via an app or smart home system. You can use your smart home setup to trigger red lights to gradually kick in automatically as evening begins. Specific red spectrum light has been scientifically linked to increased blood flow, collagen production, testosterone production and rejuvenation. Low level laser therapy used in certain clinics use red light lasers to address problems like hair loss and joint pain. Your focus should be to use red light as an approach to addressing sleep problems. Many smart home systems also allow setting alarms with smart bulbs. Instead of using a regular, jarring alarm clock to wake you up every morning, you can trigger the smart lights to wake you up with red lights that brighten and eventually turn blue to wake you up.

The moment you wake up, the most powerful way you can begin your day is to expose your entire body to natural sunlight for at least 10 minutes. Yes, I am suggesting that you take your clothes off when you do this. You will feel better, balance your vitamin D levels and allow the receptors in your cells to awaken. You will quickly notice that this one activity is as good as having a strong cup of coffee. Use light to your advantage and hack your sleeping habits.

Sound Sleep: Pay attention to the sound present in your sleep environment. If your bedroom features a noisy neighbor or poor sound damping, investing in a few decent acoustic sound absorbing panels will really help. Acoustic panels are available for home studios and the more recent variants allow beautiful, aesthetic designs so that your bedroom does not have to feature ugly walls. Acoustic panels also are generally the size of a painting and work well in damping sound without requiring your bedroom to look like a recording studio with wall to wall sound dampening foam. My bedroom has ended up looking great while isolating a lot of sound from outside thanks to these panels. I've actually had a friend ask me where I got my unique 'artwork' on my walls from. The goal with this sleep environment hack is not to create a room that looks aesthetically like you're on a space station but to prevent external noises from jarring you out of sleep. If you are using a humidifier and a good air purifier, you will already have a decent amount of white noise in your room. White noise is any type of hissing, humming or sustained intensity sound. In a sleep context if used correctly, white noise can be used to entrain your brain into a state of beautiful, restful sleep with pleasant dreams. Air conditioners, air purifiers and refrigerators on their own provide white noise that could be relaxing although some people find the constant hum of something in the room annoying. In order to really amplify the quality of your sleep using white noise, I recommend getting a white noise machine. Like most devices, you can pick these devices up ranging from $ 20 to over a $ 100 but the basic functionality is for the device to generate tones and sounds that are relaxing. Many of these devices feature natural forest sounds, swooshing waves and other sounds like isochronic tones that can have an incredible impact on your sleep. When paired with good room sound dampening, you will be amazed at the impact on your sleep. White noise generators are also a good option for those who want to use an air purifier but are annoyed by the sound of it. You don't even have to spend money on a device. There are plenty of tones and recorded sounds available on iTunes and Youtube to help you sleep but I recommend a dedicated white noise machine over those options because it would incline you to leave your devices like laptops and tablets outside your bedroom at bedtime.

Technique 6: Auto-suggestion & Mental Sleep Hacks

Auto suggestion is a technique used to self-hypnotize yourself into positive mindsets. I cannot oversell this incredibly simple and powerful technique to change just about anything in your that needs changing. Affirmations are a comparable technique but auto-suggestion takes it to the next level. The idea is to formulate a statement the same way you would form an affirmation statement meaning it has to be a statement that is positive and believable. You will then repeat your auto-suggestion to yourself a few times just before you fall asleep while you are in bed. This is a key element because the short window of time that you are in bed about to fall asleep is also your most suggestible time period when your mind is open to hypnotic suggestion.

An example of a statement that can be used to address a sleep problem would be "I love to sleep on time and I will have quality and timely sleep tonight." Try to use words that are conversationally used by you. Write it down on a post it note next to your bed to remind you to actually do the auto-suggestion. You can repeat the suggestion 20 times if possible but if you fall asleep before you have said the suggestion 20 times, that is alright and in fact a good problem to have. If you manage to state the auto suggestion 20 times and are still not asleep, that is still ok. Just know that with each practice of auto-suggestion you are programming yourself deeply and a time will come when the behavior you are trying to modify will change effortlessly and automatically. It is common to have your mind wander during the auto-suggestion practice and that is also perfectly acceptable. Just go with the flow of thoughts and gently move back to continuing the auto-suggestion practice. As you can tell, auto-suggestion can be used to combat any bad habit or thought process that isn't serving you. Just work on structuring the auto-suggestion statement effectively and keep the faith as you practice for as long as you can. Treating auto-suggestion as a daily activity before sleeping can help anchor your practice to sleeping when you begin programming yourself which is a very positive stimulus response routine.

A common symptom noticed in insomniacs is clock watching. The anxiety of watching a clock progress through the night while you lay in bed will create a negative feedback loop that will keep you awake. Getting rid of clocks from your bedroom can help greatly. Of course, this means you can still check your phone. Aside from mentally preventing yourself from picking up your phone in the middle of the night, use the technique mentioned earlier about using apps to restrict phone usage at bed time.

Technique 7: Sleep Supplements that won't turn you into a zombie

Modern medicine has surprisingly few options to enable good sleep. Sleep medication has claimed the life of many a celebrity and you should be concerned if you rely on sleeping pills to sleep. I'm going to list some supplements that can really help improve your sleep without turning you into a junkie.

- **Magnesium:** Magnesium is very important in many enzymatic reactions and is unfortunately found in dwindling quantities in US soil thanks to modern agriculture techniques. Forms of Magnesium are commonly prescribed for bone related health but commonly overlooked is its ability to relieve insomnia. They are easy to procure because they are not addictive. The best forms of magnesium tend to end with the letters 'ate'. Read the label for these letters before buying a Magnesium Supplement. Magnesium Oxide therefore is not a great choice as a sleep supplement. Magnesium Citrate however would be a better form. In some people, Magnesium can have mild stimulant effects so it's best to experiment or ask a medical professional about supplementing. Finding the right form of Magnesium for you would be worth it because it would easily improve your sleep quality in addition to all the other benefits like bone health. Epsom salts used to calm upset stomachs also tend to have a high magnesium content but rather than consuming Epsom salts, try soaking your feet in warm water with Epsom salts about an hour before bedtime.

- **Activated charcoal:** Charcoal tablets have the ability to detox the body. People usually use activated charcoal supplements to help cope with gut and stomach related ailments like Celiac disease but an often overlooked hack is to use activated charcoal tablets to improve sleep. Charcoal helps act as a heavy metal detoxing agent and absorbs toxins created by your gut bacteria. These toxins can interfere with brain chemistry optimal for sleep. Popping one or two charcoal tablets at bedtime could lead to more restful sleep and more importantly help you feel more refreshed without any of the dependency issues associated with conventional sleeping pills. I use activated charcoal tablets on nights when I anticipate a shorter sleep window or when I've travelled to a place in a different time zone. There are however things to be kept in mind when it comes to taking charcoal supplements regularly. Charcoal supplements can impact absorption of nutrients and induce constipation in some cases. It's best to not take charcoal supplements every day but use it as an adjunct therapy on nights when you cannot sleep or expect a smaller duration of sleep. Charcoal supplements also absorb certain nutrients from your body like Vitamin C so it would be prudent to supplement with Vitamin C the day after you have taken a charcoal supplement.

- **Collagen:** One of the best sleep hacks involves supplementing collagen at bedtime. Take it about 45 minutes before you go to bed and you will see an improvement in the quality of your sleep. The other benefit of taking collagen at bedtime is its ability to reverse some signs of aging, including dry skin and wrinkles. The sleep effects induced by collagen are mild and unlike conventional sleeping pills will improve your sleep without causing drowsiness the next day or building a dependency in you. You don't need a prescription and there are many options to obtain collagen supplements usually boosted with additional vitamin C. Bulletproof collagen is the brand I recommend as a drink before bedtime but there are many good supplements that will get the job done. Pill forms are also available if you are not up for drinking something before bedtime.

- **Fish oil:** We've heard enough about fish oil being good for things like joint inflammation, eyesight and muscle repair. Using forms of fish oil like Krill oil in conjunction with supplements like collagen will allow a synergistic boost to your sleep quality.

These are the more unconventional supplements to help you sleep better but I've left out the more mainstream approaches including Chamomile tea, Passionflower tea and Valerian root supplements either because I consider them as mainstream sleep supplements. Valierian also can have the opposite effect on some people so definitely check with your Doctor about starting a natural supplement regimen. I'll be going into more ways to hack your sleep quality using non habit forming supplements on sleepquation.com.

Technique 8: Visualize & Succeed

A lot has been said about the power of visualization. We already intuitively understand that visualizing a certain outcome can improve the odds of that outcome being realized. If elite athletes can use visualization techniques to improve their game, bedtime procrastinators and insomniacs can also utilize visualization to address their sleep patterns. Your mind automatically creates images all the time and its time you began to use this mechanism to your advantage. The key is to start associating positive imagery and sensations with your early bedtime routine while creating awareness within yourself of tangible consequences. The way to use this technique is to spend a few minutes every day for at least a week visualizing outcomes. A structured visualization exercise for beating bedtime procrastination is outlined below and yes it is identical to the exercise performed when writing in your sleep journal. Do it at least once a day for 7 days in addition to entries in your sleep journal to see results:

1. Imagine the effect that bedtime procrastination is having on your life – physically, mentally and spiritually. See how this habit is negatively affecting you and what that impact would be 5 years from now. You would see yourself sluggish, aging faster, losing out on opportunities, seeing others overtake you in their lives' progress, etc. This visualization will cause some pain but that's the idea. Do this step for at least a minute or for a couple of minutes.

2. Take a break and disassociate from what you saw in step one. Shake it out, stand up, wash your face and take a short break.

3. Don't take too long a break in step 2 and get back to the positive part of your visualization. See yourself conquering your bedtime procrastination and insomnia, sleeping soundly and deeply, waking up refreshed and productive every day. Start projecting your visions into the future where you see yourself achieving all your goals and winning at life in every arena. Experience the joy of sleeping regularly and consistently for many years. How will you feel? How will you look? Don't you think you would achieve more in life? Have fun with this one and if possible spend more time on this step than you spent on step 1. Project your positive vision 10

years into the future to really form a clear picture of what the long term implications are from sleeping well and eliminating your sleep procrastination habit.

Don't let the simplicity of visualization fool you. It's extremely powerful and in the long run you will see changes with regular practice even if you relapse and sleep late for a day or two or through a weekend for instance. To amplify and catalyze your progress, also work towards allowing the appropriate visualization to creep into the sleep environment preparation stage. A simple hack to further amplify your sleep potential and regularity is to ensure that your bedroom features items and cues mostly to sleeping well. This means eliminating distracting anchors and cues like television sets from your bedroom. In order to aide your visualization exercises, place pictures in your bedroom that relate to sleep. Some clients have had a lot of fun picking out art works that featured images of people sleeping soundly. One client who had tremendous trouble sleeping had pictures of babies and animals sleeping artfully displayed on his walls along with a framed print of Salvadore Dali's 'Sleep' artwork. This further conditions your mind to respect the act of sleeping so that your entire system can learn to appreciate this contrasting opposite state to the rest of your active busy day.

Technique 9: Controlling Dopamine Production

Late night binge behavior that causes sleep procrastination can be a result of an overdose of dopamine, the brain chemical associated with the pleasure center of our brain. People with addictions will usually have higher levels of dopamine in their brain. This technique for addressing your sleep issues involves identifying and fixing addictive pattern behavior. Many people are addicted to things that are not necessarily substance related. You could be addicted to TV shows or Youtube or video games or online porn or social media. Those patterns then affect your dopamine production levels to the point where your sleep patterns get affected. This is particularly relevant in cases where the sufferer feels puzzled about their own inability to go to bed on time while they were watching TV for instance. Since dopamine regulates the pleasure center of the brain, addressing its natural production cycle will also allow your bad habits to be eliminated. When you indulge in addictive behavior that involves persistently elevated dopamine levels, the brain reacts by shutting down the number of available receptors for dopamine. This is why chronic sleep procrastinators have such a hard time sticking to a new routine once adopted. The consistent night time dopamine rush someone experiences from consuming online porn for instance will inevitably have a negative follow on effect on sleep. Think about it – your cave person brain would instinctively choose an activity related to sex than sleep if it had a choice. It will be difficult to only use willpower to bulldoze through a bad habit. Sleep procrastinators face a compounded challenge because lack of sleep is directly tied to lower willpower.

The good news is that if you are able to abstain from a harmful activity or bad habit, your brain's dopamine receptors will also increase and in time you will not be addicted to Netflix, porn, etc. Your highs will be more regulated and controllable. Improving your sleep will further increase your motivation and willpower allowing you to sustain your progress in life.

The first step in managing dopamine production to support optimal sleep patterns is to honestly evaluate your night time routine and identify any behaviors that resemble addictive patterns. If you find yourself checking Facebook every night and spending hours on end, that would be your identified habit to change. Once you are aware of the habits that could be impacting your dopamine production regulation, start making changes to your routine or mechanically prevent yourself from indulging in the activity. I've outlined methods to control access to digital devices so that you may not indulge in them after a specific time. Identify the cues that lead you down the path to engaging in the bad habit. You might notice someone checking their phone and feel a sudden urge to check your Facebook shortly thereafter (assuming that you have a social media addiction).

Once you have a good idea of the patterns of behavior to address in order to alleviate your bedtime procrastination, it's a good idea to begin a regular mindfulness practice. Mindfulness has shown enormous potential in helping drug addicts and alcoholics so this is a practice worth investing time into. It's far from rocket science and essentially involves becoming aware of the sensations related to the urge or habit. You can begin by paying attention to how your breathing and sensations in your body changed as the urge to watch yet another Game of Thrones episode increased for instance. I highly recommend picking up a copy of "The Power of Now" by

Eckhart Tolle if you haven't already. There are a number of books on being in the moment and the 'Now' series is a great way to get into general mindful living that will positively impact all areas of your life. I love consuming this content in audiobook format and highly recommend using the audiobook versions of the Now series to meditate. You will feel so centered and grounded that your impulse control muscles will grow significantly stronger in as short a time as a few weeks of practice. This can be thought of as brain training to help you better recognize the gap between stimulus and response. By paying mindful attention to your internal state laced with curiosity, you might discover a more hidden pain or anxiety causing your bedtime procrastination or insomnia. One of my clients for instance had a very superficial and small set of friends. His bedtime procrastination was a result of a sense of loneliness. Addressing his social issues led to an improvement in his general sleep routine.

A more complex topic related to self-control even in sleep related schedules relates to whether or not you have an undiagnosed case of Asperger's or ADHD. If you suspect you have symptoms that match Asperger's, OCD or ADD disorders, it would be worth consulting with a qualified therapist to get a diagnosis. Addressing the broader psychological issue would further impact your sleep procrastination and insomnia issues.

Putting it all together – Conclusion

You should approach your tendency to procrastinate your bedtime in a similar manner that a long time smoker tries to quit smoking. You are an addict to this type of behavior so the key to beating addiction is to remain consistent in your efforts to correcting your sleep habits. You are compulsively sleeping late on a regular basis because deep down your internal value set probably allows you to do so. Reflection in general and journaling should allow you to understand your values and figure out why you don't think appropriate sleep times are important to you. If you don't think sleeping late on a consistent basis is ok, then you would be far less likely to indulge in it. Think about whether you think there's little wrong in when you go to bed late every night. You might consciously know that sleeping late causes distress the next day, upsets your schedule, keeps you from achieving the things you want to achieve and has you groggy for most of the following day. Unconsciously however, your values might not align with that and imagine living your entire life with this conflict embedded within you. That's why it's extremely important to understand your own values and how they align with your behaviors. The odds are that since you picked up this book, you most likely feel a need to correct his behavior. Understand that millions of people suffer from bedtime procrastination tendencies but few actually are honest with themselves about the ramifications. They rationalize it away as either a part of modern living or something that everyone has to go through. By fixing this habit, you will likely see many other problem areas of your life unravel.

Sleep is one of those areas that tend to be impacted by ancillary lifestyle factors. It's worth investing time into understanding what those underlying factors which could include the substances you consume on a daily basis (alcohol, marijuana, coffee, etc.), your sleep environment or issues from your childhood. These underlying factors would have to be addressed to reduce your sleep procrastination tendencies.

I've approached bedtime procrastination treatment options from the standpoint of eliminating bad habits and addictions that lead to procrastinated sleep schedules but it is important to note that in the minority of cases involving disrupted sleep schedules, medical causes are to blame. It's worth getting your blood work done to eliminate any underlying health factors that may be keeping you from going to bed on time or getting restful sleep.

Journaling is the one practice that I recommend for moving you towards becoming an early riser and regularizing your sleep patterns. A sleep journal is a highly underrated tool and I suggest initializing your sleep journal practice in the mornings before running through each of the techniques listed in the book. Write down your observations and in time you will become more reflective. Even though your journal is designated as a sleep journal, it's very common to gain strong insights in other areas of your life. Do not ignore these insights and try to further slice this new information to understand if there is a linkage to your disrupted sleep tendencies. You can absolutely eliminate this issue in your life if you choose to do so. Remember: mastering your sleep is mastering your life. You were drawn to this book because your intention to sleep well has crystallized. It is now time to channel this intention into reality. Never ever give up. People are not born night owls or early birds. The choice is yours.

If you thought this book had ideas that you hadn't heard before and it helped you overcome your bedtime procrastination or insomnia let me know at <u>sleepquation.com,</u> the blog that I write for. Do leave a review for this book on Amazon. I hope the effort placed in researching and identifying unique ideas has shone through in this book. Go to bed now!

Dylan's other work

Fast Motivation That Lasts - Check out Dylan Johnson's work on re-igniting motivational energy. It contains powerful techniques and ideas to help you reinvigorate your life. ASIN: B01N2AB4Y4

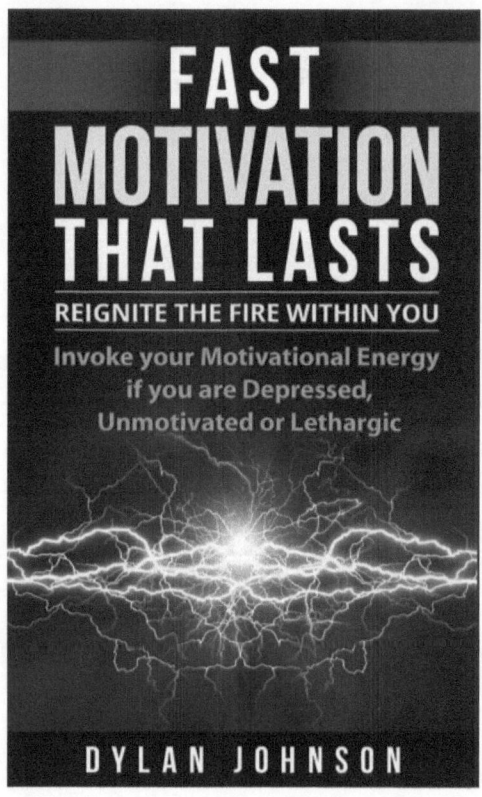

Ultimate Fitness Mindset – the "inner game" of fitness. Dylan's exploration of techniques to stay fit using the power of the mind to lose weight, stay fit and consistent with healthy habits. ASIN: B01MYHDQGM

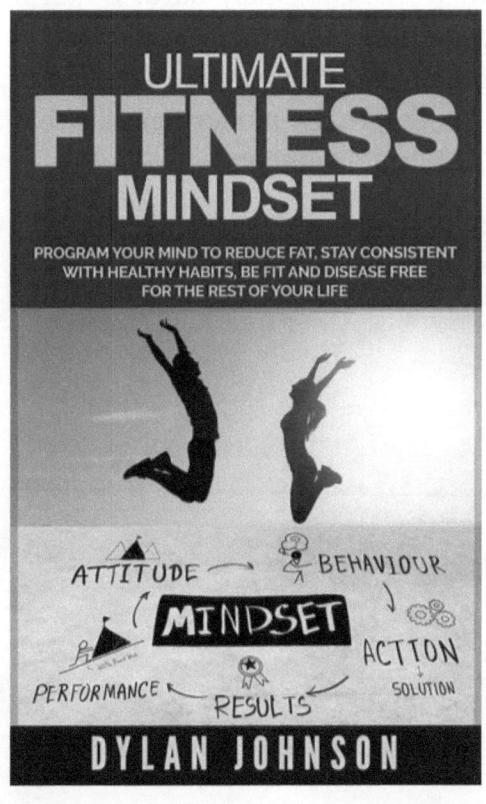

Mind of Musk – Elon Musk is one of the few individuals in the world today who has made bold, optimistic predictions about the future and then gone on to actually execute towards them. We admire him because he is sincere, takes big bets and works extremely hard. Dylan has gone into incredible depth beyond the standard biography to come up with actionable insights on how to think like the modern genius that is Elon Musk. ASIN: 1521993637

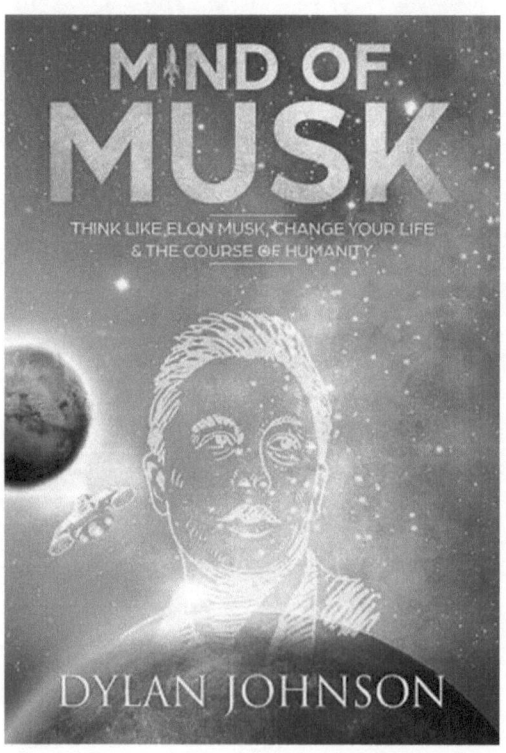